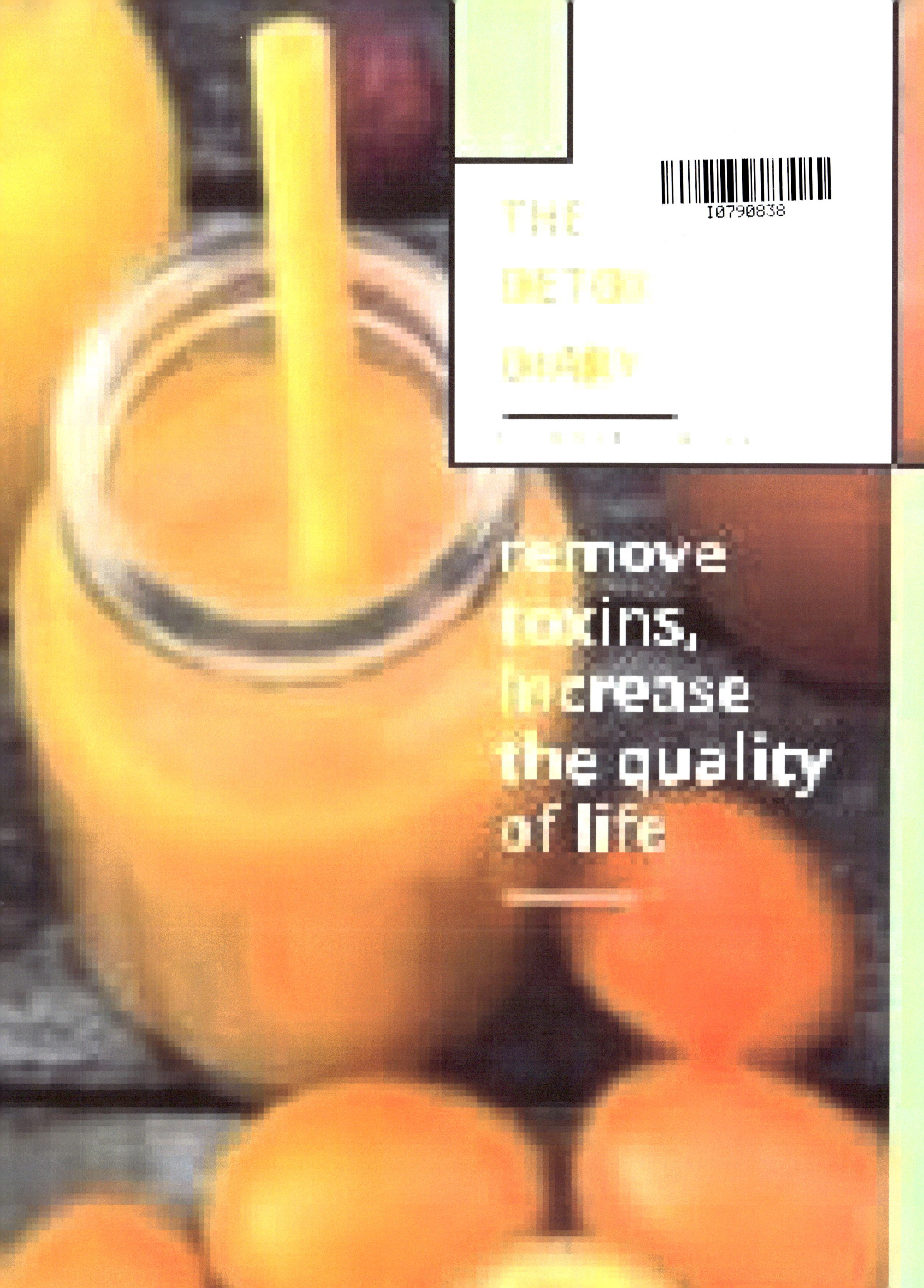
I0790838
THE
DETOX
DIARY
remove
toxins,
increase
the quality
of life

The Detox Diary: Disconnect to Connect Vol. 1

Lucid Press

10355 South Jordan Gateway

Ste. 300

South Jordan, UT 84095

www.lucidpress.com

The information and solutions offered in this resource are a result of years of study, research, and practical life application. These intended guidelines are not to replace professional medical advice or counseling. ALIA D. WALTHALL and RESTORATION IS POSSIBLE make no warranties, representations, or guarantees regarding any particular result or outcome. Any and all express or implied warranties are disclaimed. For individual conditions and needs, please consult qualified medical and psychological services.

ALIA D. WALTHALL and RESTORATION IS POSSIBLE do not condone treating yourself, or any other person, disclaim any and all liability arising directly or indirectly from the information in this resource. For more information on RESTORATION IS POSSIBLE, email guidedtolight@gmail.com.

Printed in the United States of America.

7861697

ISBN-13: 978-1981332502

ISBN-10: 1981332502

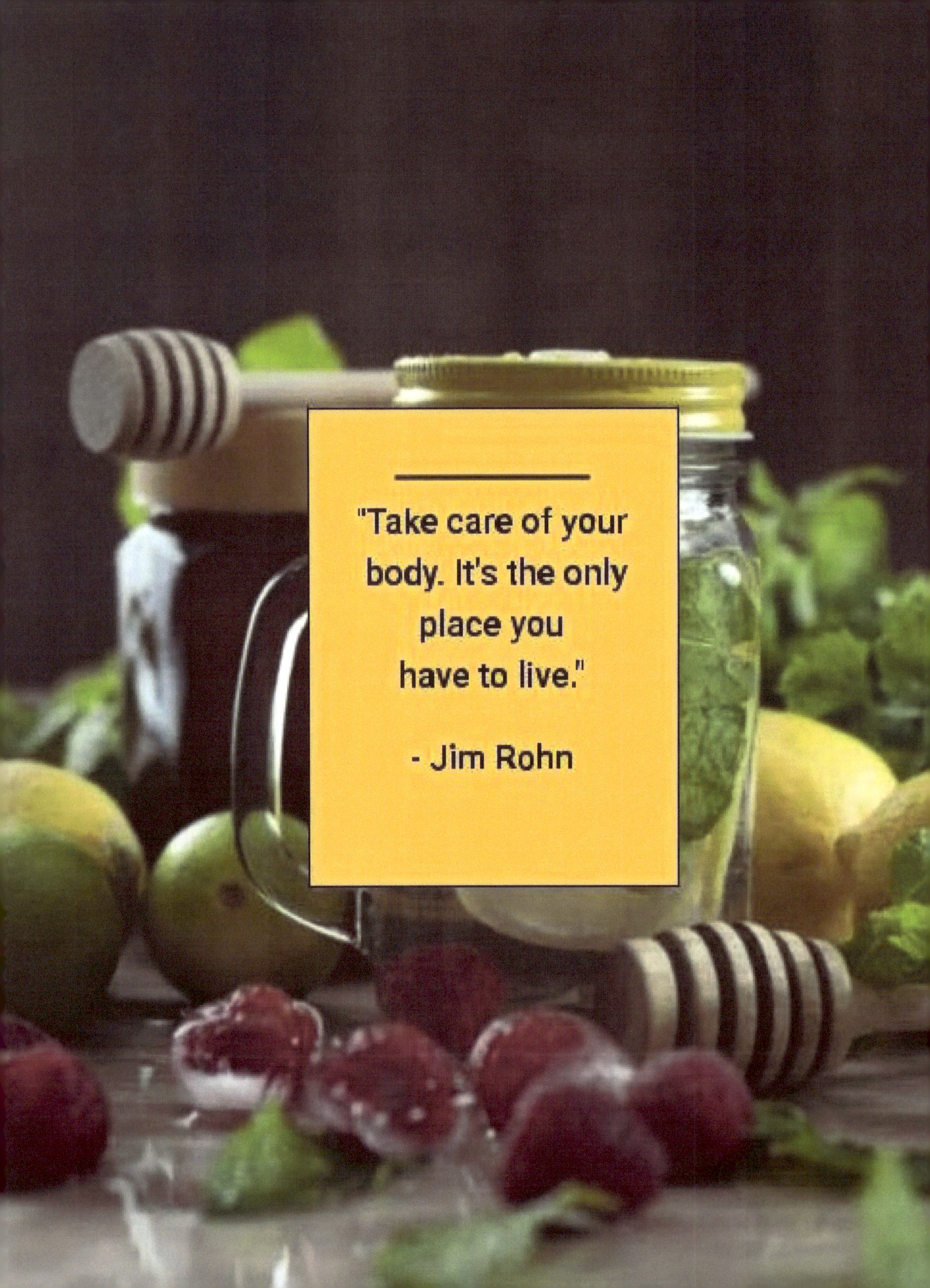

"Take care of your body. It's the only place you have to live."

- Jim Rohn

ABOUT THE AUTHOR

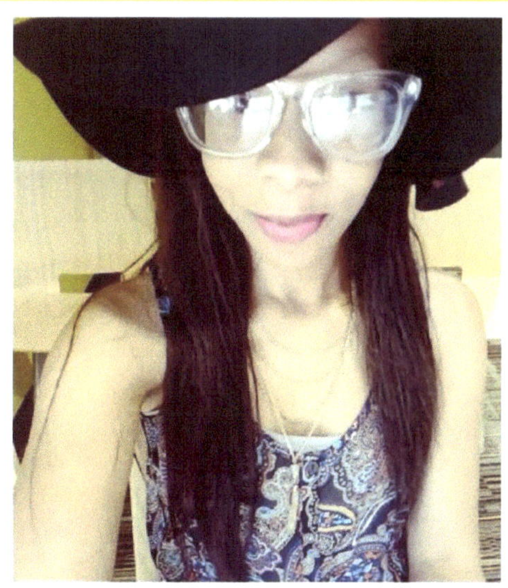

Alia D. Walthall holds a Bachelor of Arts in Psychology from the University of Memphis, and has extensive knowledge in holistic health and remedies, EFT/Body Code, Chromotherapy, Crystal Healing, and various other energy therapies. She is the sole founder of a generous company, Restoration Is Possible, and actively strives for the betterment of the mind, body, and soul.

FACEBOOK: @yourguidetolight

INSTAGRAM: @yourguidetolight

TABLE OF CONTENT

DEFINITIONS

AILMENT - an illness

CLEANSE - an attempt to rid the body of substances regarded as toxic or unhealthy typically by consuming only water or other liquids

DETOX - abstain from or rid the body of toxic or unhealthy substances

HOLISTIC HEALTH - an emphasis on the connection between mind, body, and spirit

SELF-CARE - identifying and nurturing one's individual needs

TOP REASONS TO DETOX

- Remove toxins from the body
- Prevent chronic disease
- Enhance immune system function
- Lose weight
- Slow premature aging
- Improve quality of life
- Increase energy
- Improve skin quality
- Mental and emotional clarity
- Restore balance to your body's systems

HELPFUL HINTS

While detoxing has its major benefits, and is becoming widely accepted, it is not for everyone. Two of the most important tasks are figuring out the reason(s) you need to detox, and what process works specifically for you.

IS THIS RIGHT FOR ME?

As detoxing becomes more mainstream and widely accepted, it is common to hear about the neighbor next door who lost a few pounds while detoxing - or the coworker whose skin looks more vibrant after a cleanse. As much as a detox can benefit the body, it can also cause harmful and uncomfortable symptoms when carried out improperly.

Many times we only hear of the positive effects of a detox or cleanse: more energized, less depressed, noticeable weight loss, dissipated cravings, reduced allergens, etc. However, other symptoms such as moodiness, fatigue, headache, constipation, overindulging, dizziness, etc may occur.

WHAT COULD HAPPEN?

Detoxing is an excellent gateway towards a healthier diet and breaking unhealthy patterns; however, it is not recommended to use a detox as a way to purge.

HELPFUL HINTS (CONT.)

Doing so may result in the body forming negative habits (e.g., binge-eating).

Additionally, the body can become weak when working out due to the lack of extra fuel needed when exercising.

HOW DO I AVOID THIS?

As previously mentioned, detoxing is not for everyone. If you suspect your body is facing the negative side of detoxing, then stop your routine. Make sure you are not eliminating too much of what your body needs, or that your cleanse has not exceeded too many days. If you have a medical condition, consult with your physician before starting a detox regime.

Keep your body hydrated by drinking at least 8 cups a day - especially before and after a detox bath or soak. Do not cut your calories below 1,000, and continue to incorporate carbs and "good-for-you" fats.

If you, or someone you know, experiences discomfort while detoxing, it is suggested to terminate the process. There may be ingredients you need to add or leave out. LISTEN TO YOUR BODY!

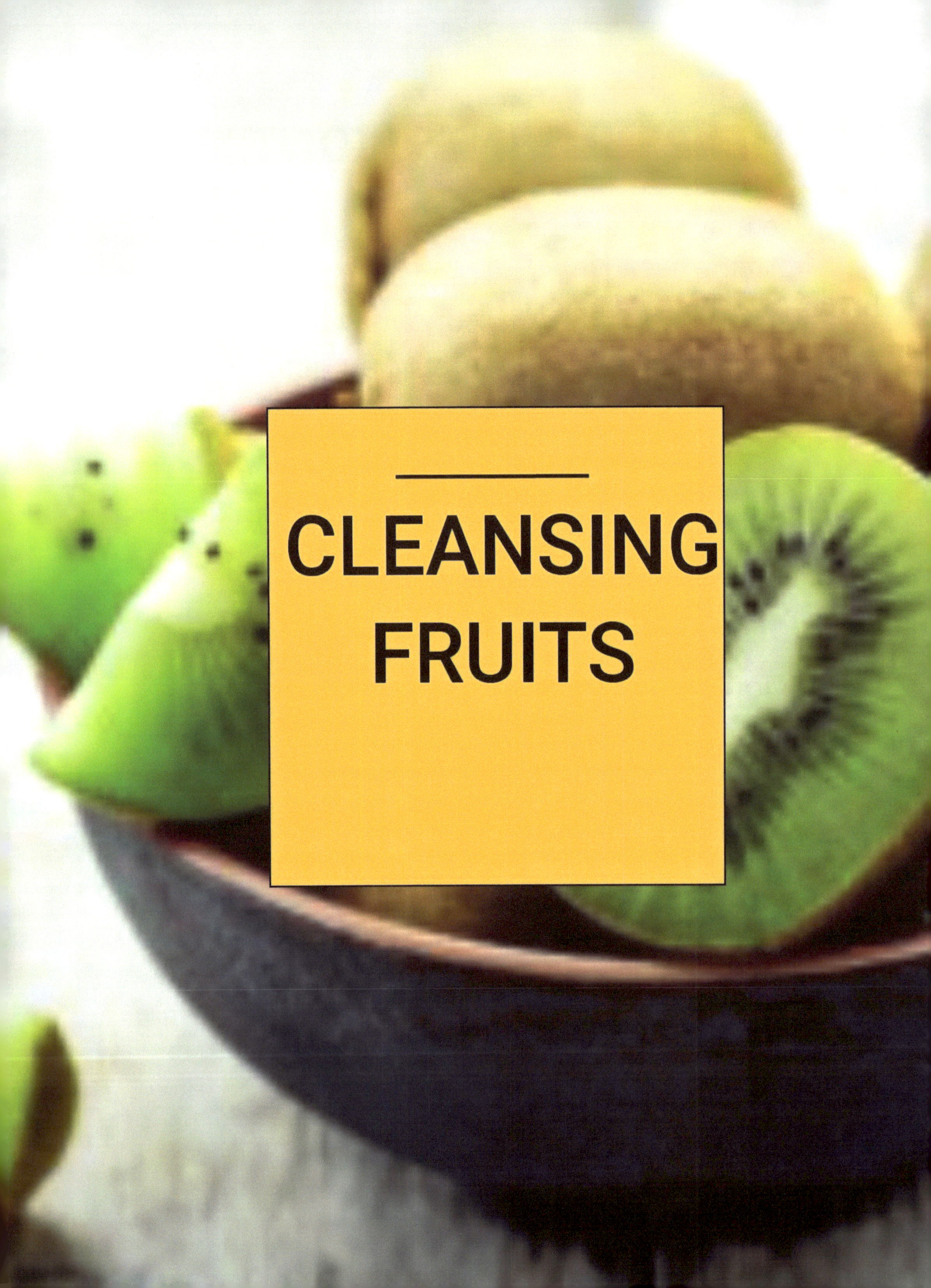

CLEANSING
FRUITS

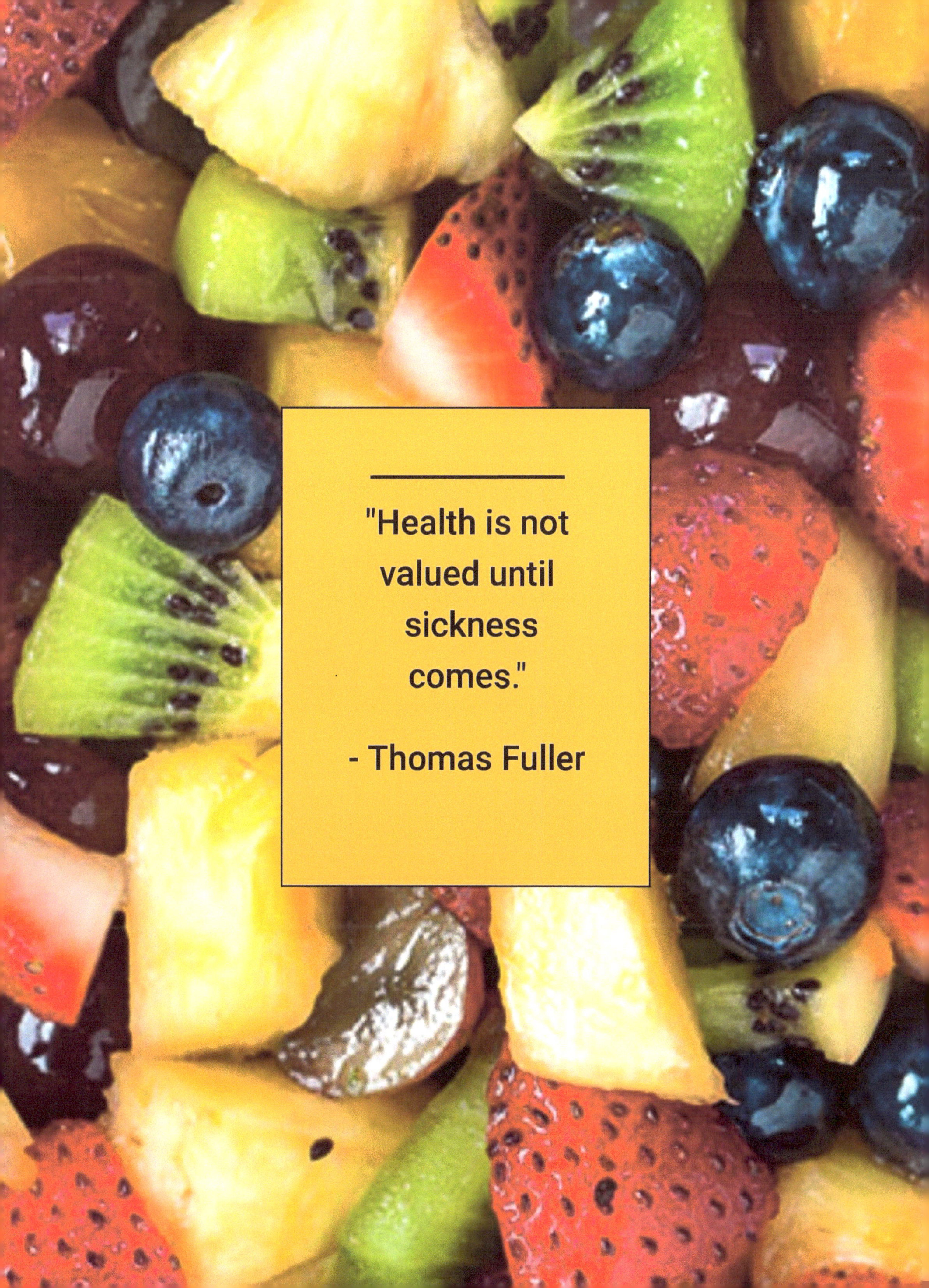

"Health is not
valued until
sickness
comes."

- Thomas Fuller

CLEANSING FRUITS

APPLES

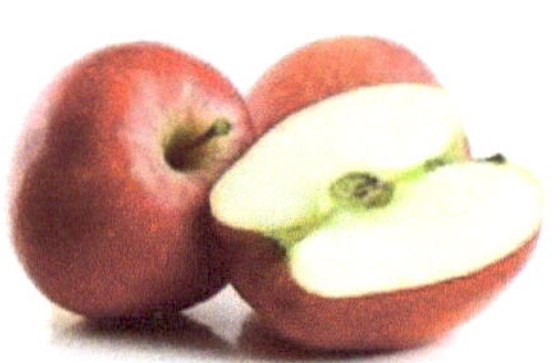

- High in pectin
- Eliminate toxic buildup
- Cleanses the intestines

AVOCADOS

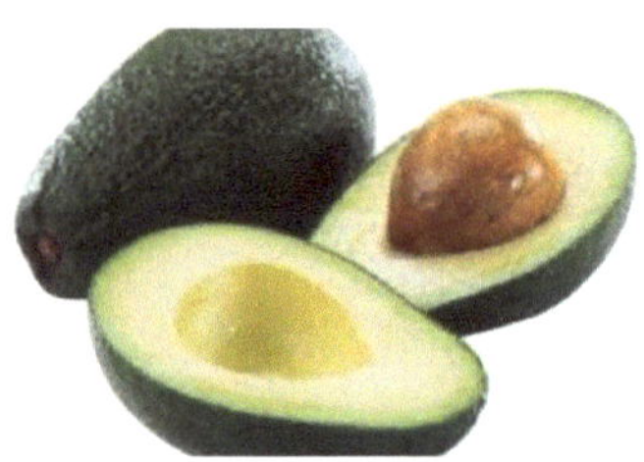

- Lowers cholesterol
- Dilates blood vessels
- Blocks toxins that destroy arteries

BLUEBERRIES

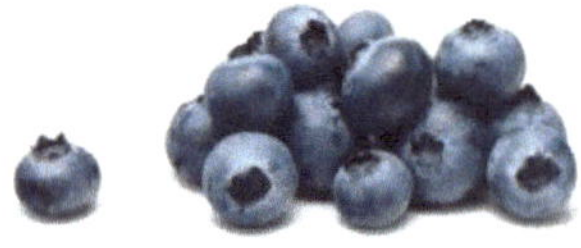

- Packed with antioxidants
- Blocks bacteria that causes Urinary Tract Infections

CRANBERRIES

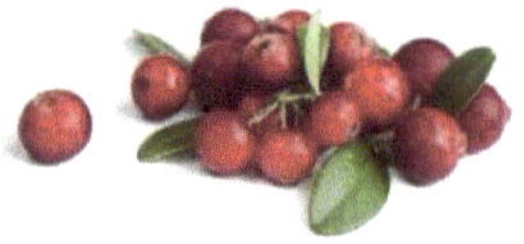

- Cleanses the body from harmful bacteria and viruses lingering in your urinary tract

CUCUMBERS

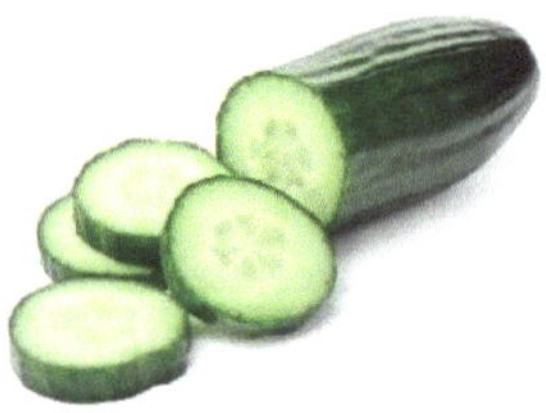

- Excellent for re-hydration

FIGS

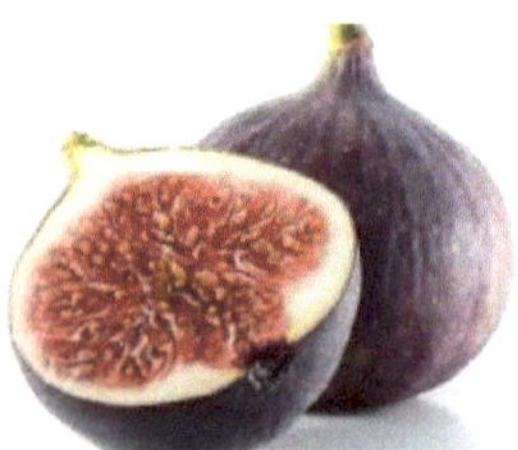

- Prevent the development of toxic urine
- Cleanses the kidney and bladder

CLEANSING FRUITS (CONT.)

GOJI BERRIES

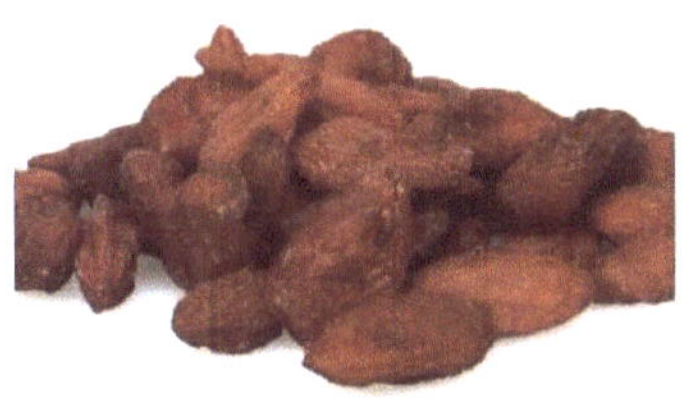

- Packs more vitamin C than oranges
- Packs more beta-carotene than carrots
- Removes waste from body
- Improves liver performance

GRAPEFRUITS

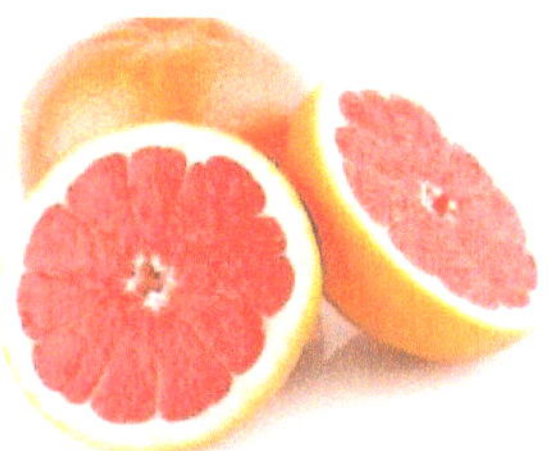

- Detoxes the liver and intestines
- Fiber rich

KIWIS

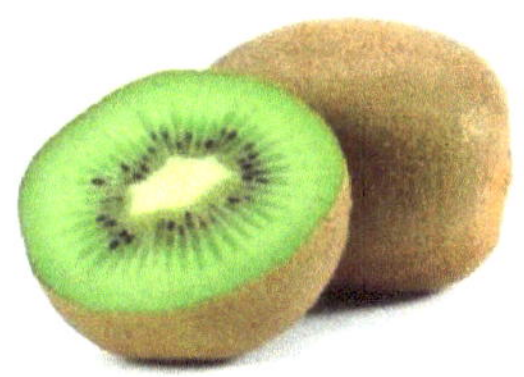

- Packed with Vitamin C
- Energy booster

LEMONS

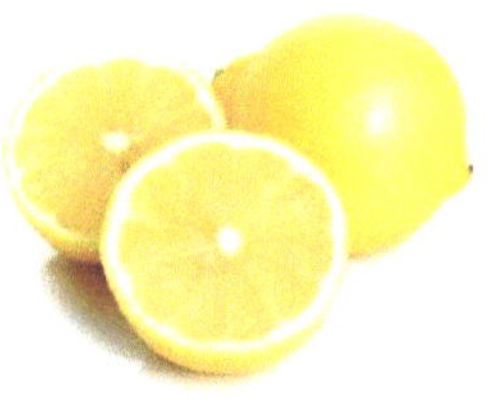

- Contains high amounts of Vitamin C
- Flushes toxins form body

PAPAYAS

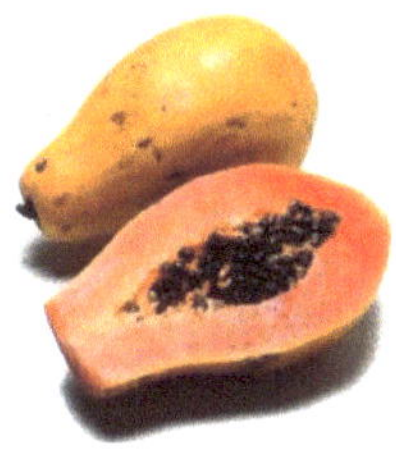

- Promotes digestive health
- Energy booster
- Detoxes the body

PINEAPPLES

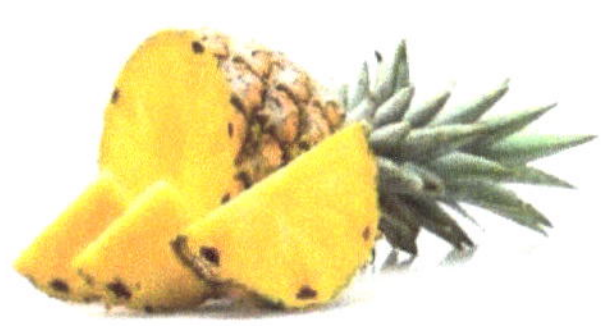

- Cleanses the colon
- Improves digestion

CLEANSING FRUITS (CONT.)

POMEGRANATES

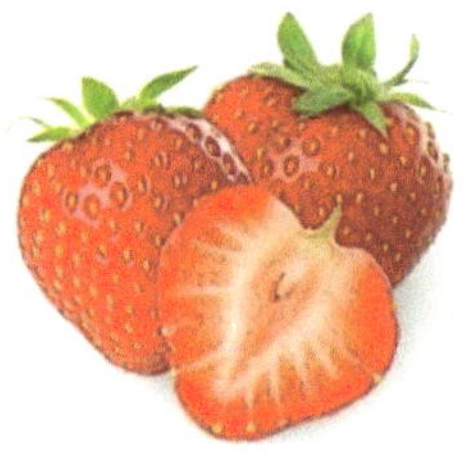

- Antioxidant boost
- Helps fight disease
- Boosts the immunie system

STRAWBERRIES

- Helps eliminate toxins
- Helps with weight loss

WATERMELON

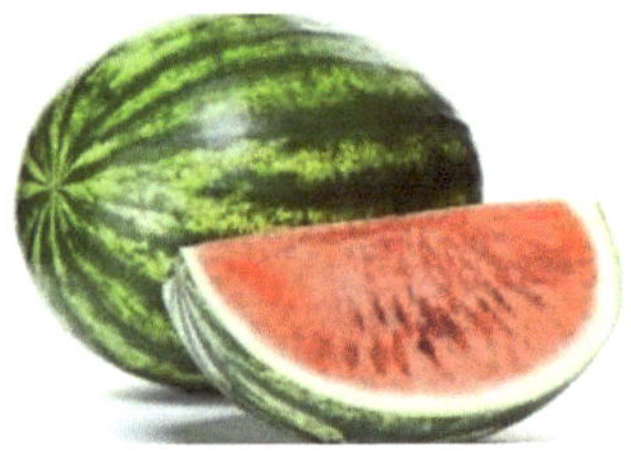

- Flushes out toxins
- Helps the liver and kidneys rid itself of ammonia

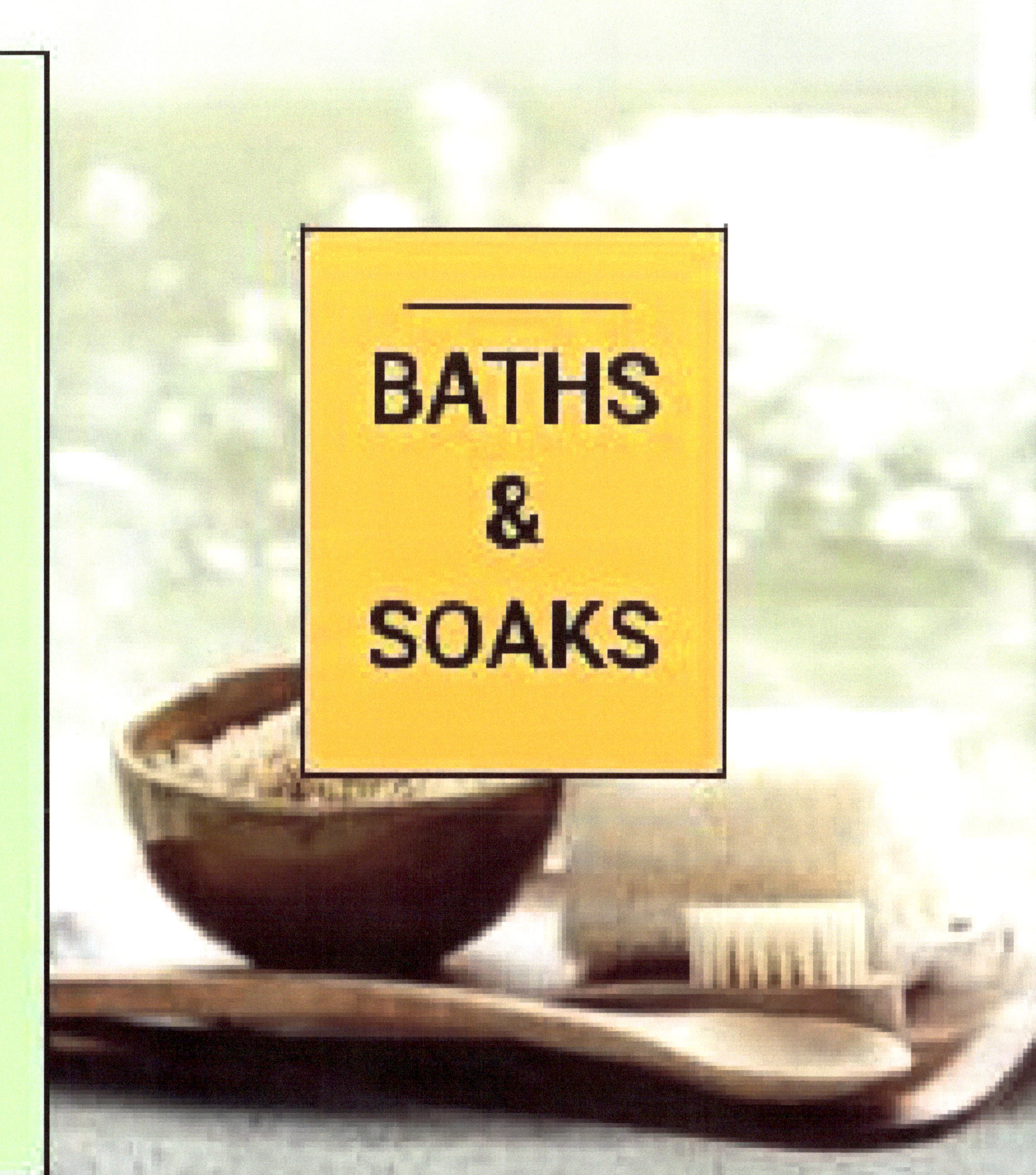
BATHS
&
SOAKS

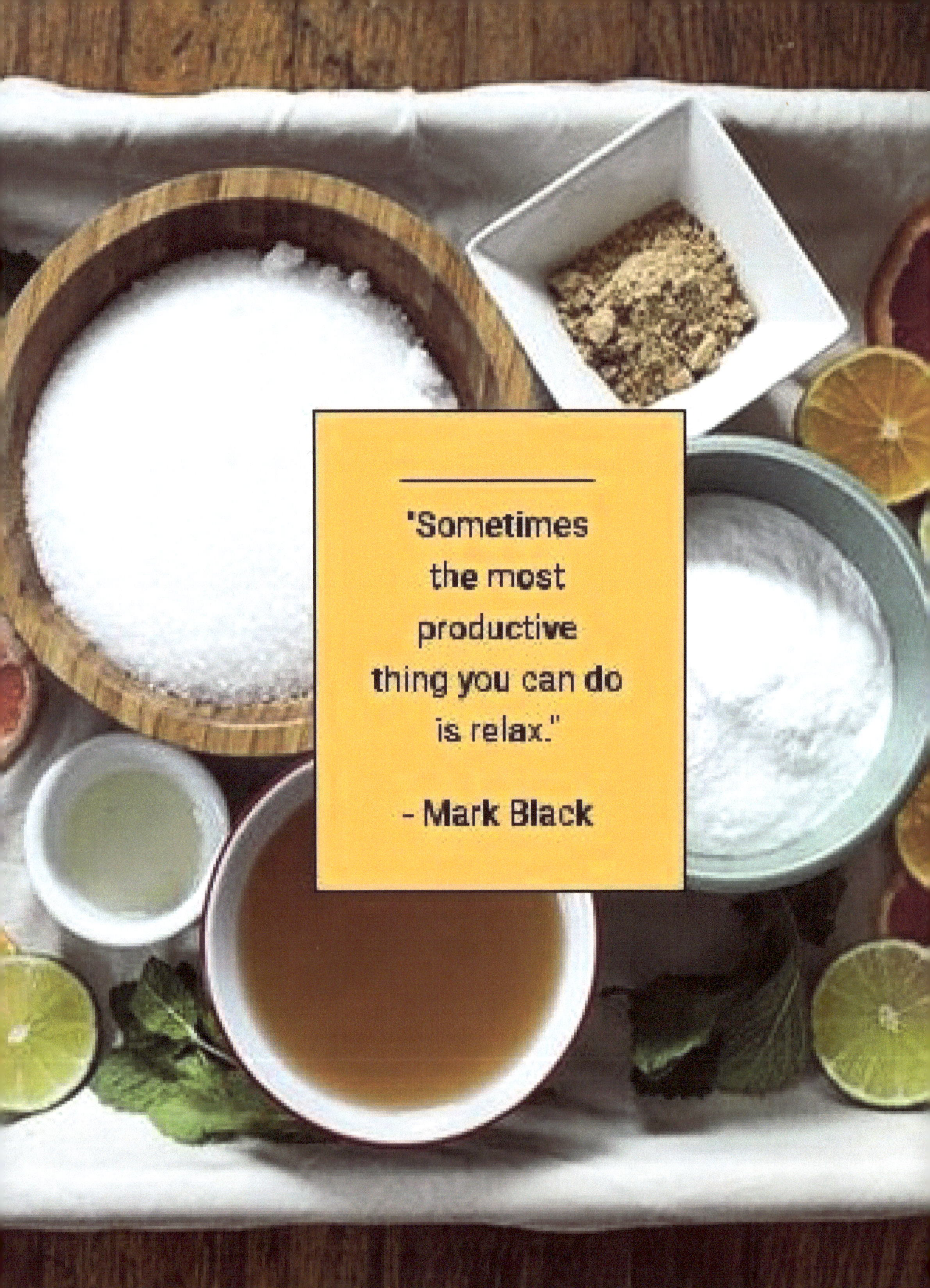
"Sometimes
the most
productive
thing you can do
is relax."

- Mark Black

BATHS & SOAKS

Salt Detox Foot Bath

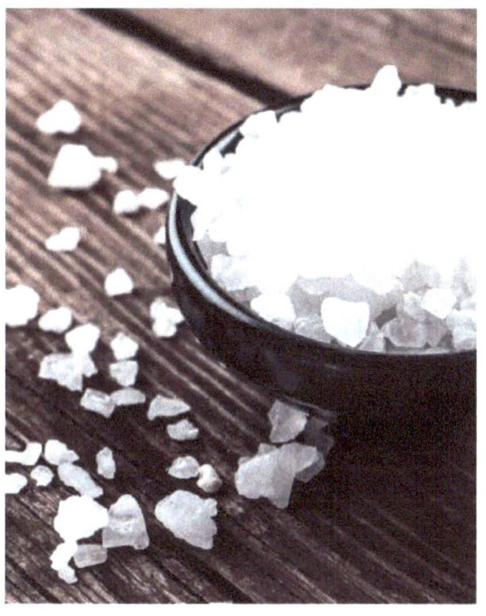

Ingredients

- 1 cup Epsom salt
- 1 cup sea salt
- 2 cups baking soda
- 1 cup apple cider vinegar
- Essential oils (optional)

Usage

- Detox the body
- Soothe skin irritation
- Increase magnesium levels

Pour boiling water in a quart size jar. Mix together the Epsom salt sea salt, and baking soda until all is dissolved. Fill a tub or bath container with warm water. Add apple cider vinegar to the tub of water, and then add the salt mixture. You may add an essential oil to this mixture. Soak your feet for 30 minutes. Exhaustion may occur.

Clay Detox Foot Bath

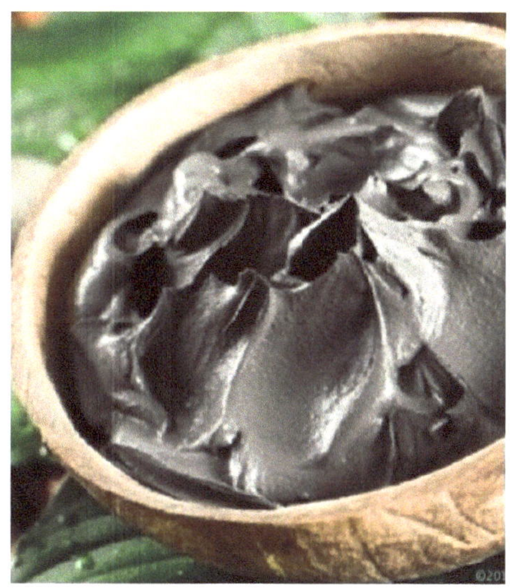

Ingredients

- 1/2 cup beentonite clay
- 1/2 cup Epsom salt
- Essential oils (optional)

Usage

- Remove toxins
- Boost magnesium levels

Pour hot water, Epsom salt, and a few drops of essential oil (optional) in a tub or bath container. Make sure you stir until all the salt is dissolved. In a separate bowl, pour some water along with the clay until you make a homogeneous paste. Add the clay paste into your soaking container, Soak your feet for at least 20 minutes.

Oxygen Detox Foot Bath

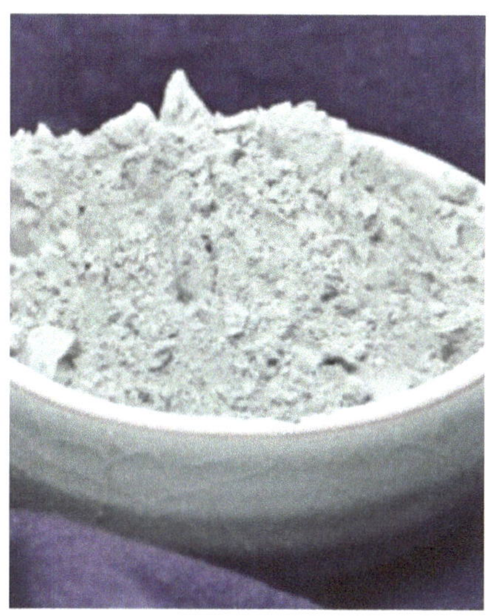

Ingredients

- 2 cups hydrogen peroxide
- 1 tablespoon dried ginger powder

Usage

- Detox the body
- Soothe pain
- Soothe skin irritation
- Soothe skin allergies

Fill a tub or bath container with hot water. Add in the dried ginger and hydrogen peroxide. Stir well, then soak your feet for 30 minutes.

*When mixing ingredients, use plastic, wooden, or glass jars and spoons.

BATHS & SOAKS (CONT.)

Green Tea Detox Bath

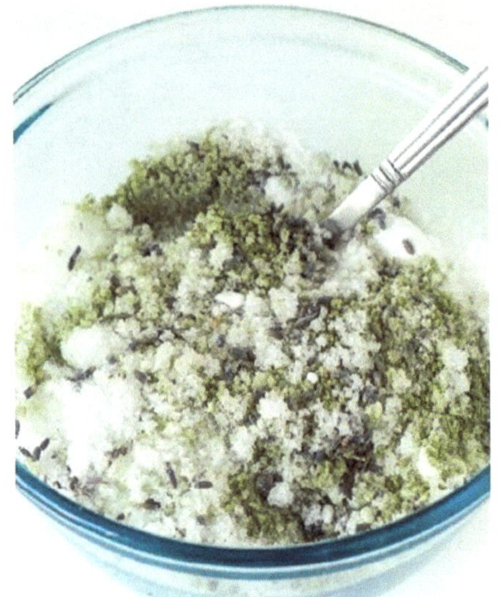

Ingredients

- 5 bags of green tea
- 1 3/4 cups of Epsom salt
- 2/3 cups of baking soda
- Essential oil (optional)

Usage

- Energy boost
- Increases antioxidant activity in the bloodstream
- Lowers cholesterol

When the tub is halfway full of water, add in all ingredients. Occasionally stir the water to make sure everything is evenly mixed and distributed. This bath can be taken anywhere from once a day to every so often. It all depends on your body's reaction.

Eucalyptus & Vanilla Bean Detox Bath

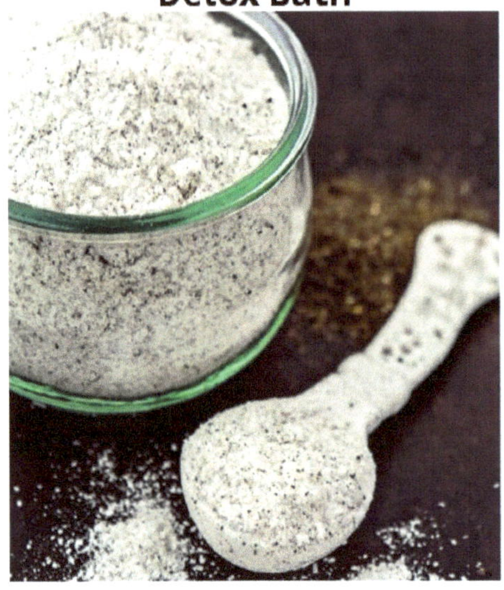

Ingredients

- 1 cup of Epsom salt
- 1/2 cup baking soda
- 3 drops of eucalyptus essential oil
- 8 drops of vanilla in jojoba oil

Usage

- Relieves dry, itchy skin
- Rids the body of toxins
- Moisturizes the skin

Make sure all ingredients are well combined in a container (preferably glass). Fill the tub halfway with warm/hot water, and add one spoonful of your detox mixture to your bath.

Ginger Detox Bath

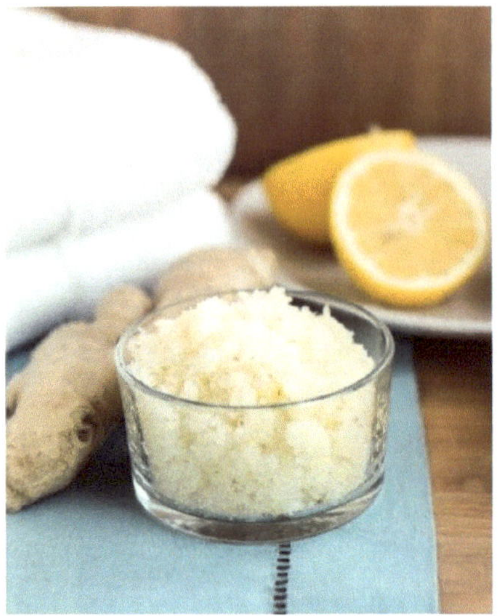

Ingredients

- 1 tablespoon of fresh ginger
- 1/2 cup of Epsom salt
- 1 tablespoon of lemon juice

Usage

- Unclogs pores
- Removes toxins from the body
- Soothes muscles

Combine ginger and 1/2 cup of Epsom salt in a a food processor until the ginger is ground. Fill the tub with warm/hot water. Place a towel down, and apply the scrub from the feet up (avoiding sensitive areas). The heat and ginger will ultimately make you sweat out the toxins.

*When mixing ingredients, use plastic, wooden, or glass jars and spoons.

BATHS & SOAKS (CONT.)

Calming Salt Detox Bath

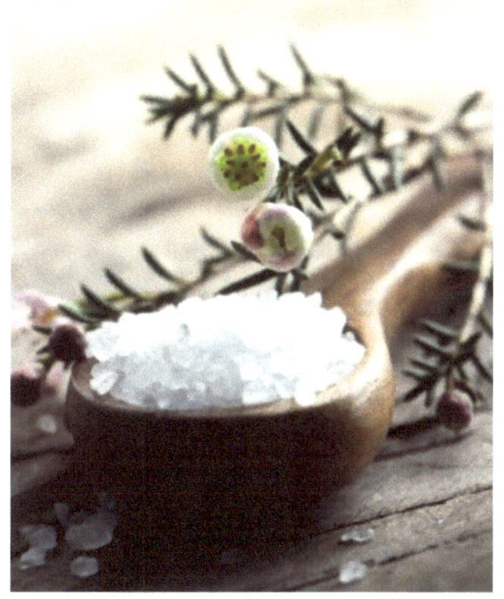

Ingredients

- 1/2 cup of Epsom salt
- 1/2 cup of real salt
- 1 1/2 cups of dead sea salt
- 1/8 cup of bentonite clay
- 7 drops of lavender essential oil
- 7 drops of frankincense essential oil

Usage

- Rids the body of toxins
- Promotes sleep
- Great for aging skin
- Relaxes the body

Add one cup of this mixture to warm/hot bath water. Soak for about 15 - 20 minutes. When rinsing off, rinse off in cold water only to close your pores.

Almond Milk Detox Bath

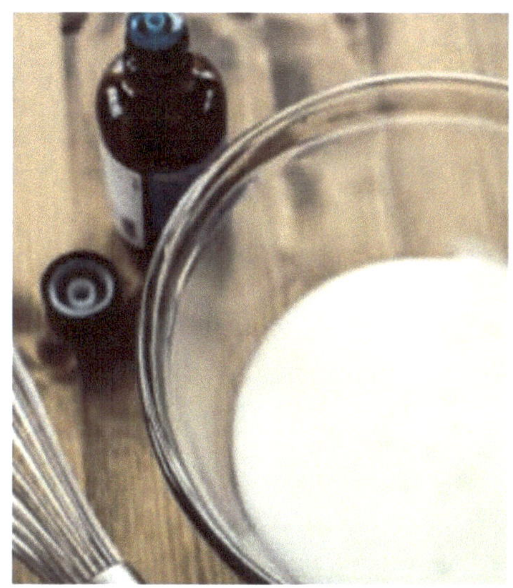

Ingredients

- 1 cup Epsom salt
- 1/2 cup baking soda
- 1/2 cup Silk Almond Milk
- 2 tablespoons of coconut oil
- 10-25 drops of essential oil (optional)

Usage

- Hydrate and soften the skin
- Relieves aches and pains
- Rich in Vitamin E
- Relaxes the body

Combine all ingredients, and add it to a warm bath while the water is still running. You may soak for about 20 - 30 minutes. If you choose, you may also pair this recipe with at least three varying essential oils.

Lemon & Rosemary Detox Bath

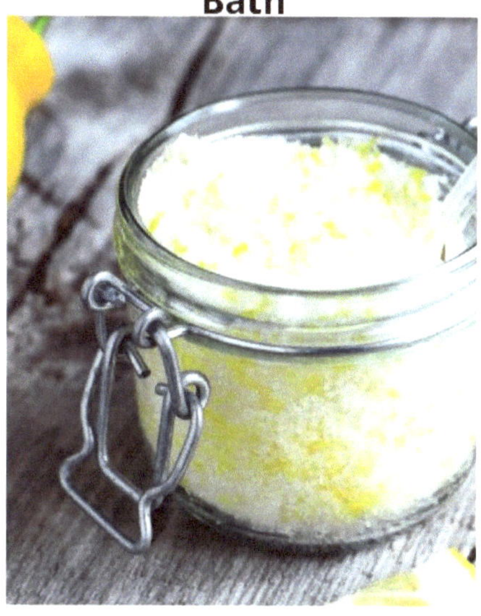

Ingredients

- 2 cups Epsom salt
- 1/2 cup baking soda
- 2-3 tablespoons of fresh rosemary
- 6-8 drops of lemon essential oil (optional)
- 2-3 tablespoons of lemon zest

Usage

- Improves memory
- Regulates the digestive system
- Soothes muscles

Combine Epsom salt and baking soda in a small bowl. Add in half of your essential oil. Mix in the chopped rosemary and lemon zest.

*When mixing ingredients, use plastic, wooden, or glass jars and spoons.

BATHS & SOAKS (CONT.)

Powdered Milk Detox Bath

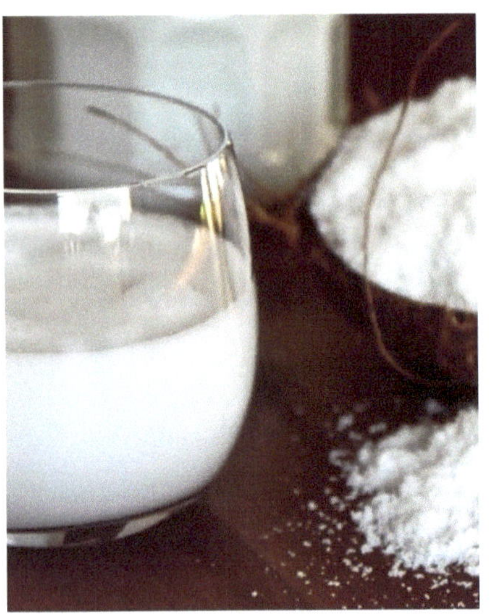

Ingredients

- 1 cup of powdered coconut milk
- 1/2 cup of baking soda
- 1/2 cup of cornstarch
- 5 - 10 drops of essential oil (optional)

Usage

- Relieves stress
- Moisturizes skin

Combine all ingredients in a glass jar (preferably a mason jar). Fill the tub with warm water, and add mixture when the water is halfway in the tub. Soak for at least 20 minutes.

Lavender Detox Bath

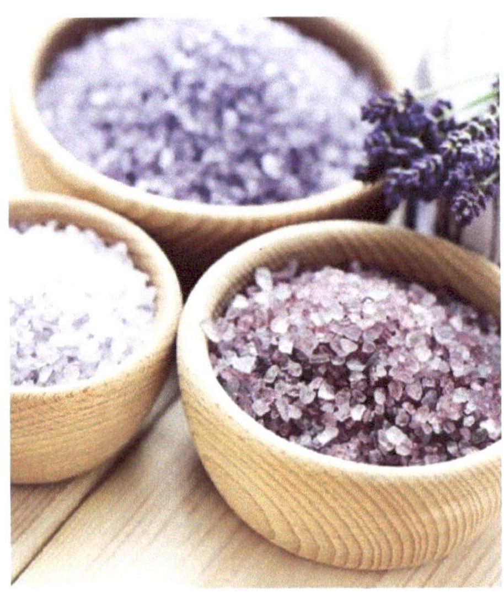

Ingredients

- 1 cup of Epsom salt
- 1 cup of baking soda
- 10 drops of lavender essential oil

Usage

- Relieves stress and soothes muscles
- Draws out toxins
- Increases the absorption of minerals

Fill the tub halfway with warm/hot water. Soak for 20 - 30 minutes. If possible, cover your entire body up to your neck. Avoid eating at least 20 minutes after you soak, and rink plenty of water.

Lavender & Eucalyptus Detox Bath

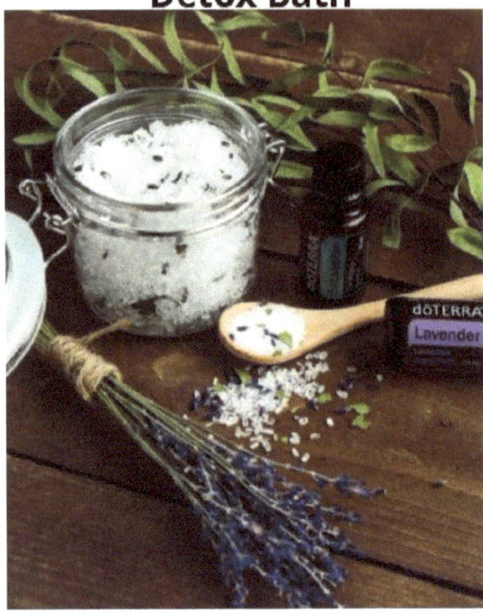

Ingredients

- 2 cups of Epsom salt
- 1/2 cup dry lavender
- 5-6 drops of lavender essential oil
- 10 drops of eucalyptus essential oil

Usage

- Treats insomnia
- Relaxes the muscles
- Relieves respiratory issues

Fill the tub halfway with very warm water. Add in ingredients. Soak for no longer then 30 minutes. Take a deep breath and emerge slowly from the tub once your bath is completed.

*When mixing ingredients, use plastic, wooden, or glass jars and spoons.

HELPFUL HINTS (CONT.)

Before you bathe:

1. Drink plenty of water to stay hydrated as toxins will soon be leaving your body.
2. Allow your body to fully digest any food intake beforehand
3. If you are testing out a new detox or are detoxing for the first time, it is suggested to have someone close by in case you experience any discomfort .

Bath prep:

1. Make sure the water temperature is hot, yet still comfortable.
2. Add ingredients when the tub is halfway full. Stir the water occasionally.
3. Soak for 20-40 minutes. Within 20 minutes, toxins begin to leave the body. The remaining 20 - 40 minutes is dedicated to allowing the minerals to be absorbed.
4. Some detoxes allow for daily use, while others allow for occasional usage. It all depends on your body's natural reaction.

After you bathe:

1. Exit the bath slowly in case you experience symptoms of dizziness or headache. Such discomfort will subside within minutes.
2. Drink plenty of water to re-hydrate yourself.
3. If needed, use olive oil. coconut oil. or other natural products to moisturize the skin.
4. Rinse off in cool water to close your pores..

If you, or someone you know, experiences discomfort while detoxing, it is suggested to terminate the process. There may be ingredients you need to add or leave out. LISTEN TO YOUR BODY!

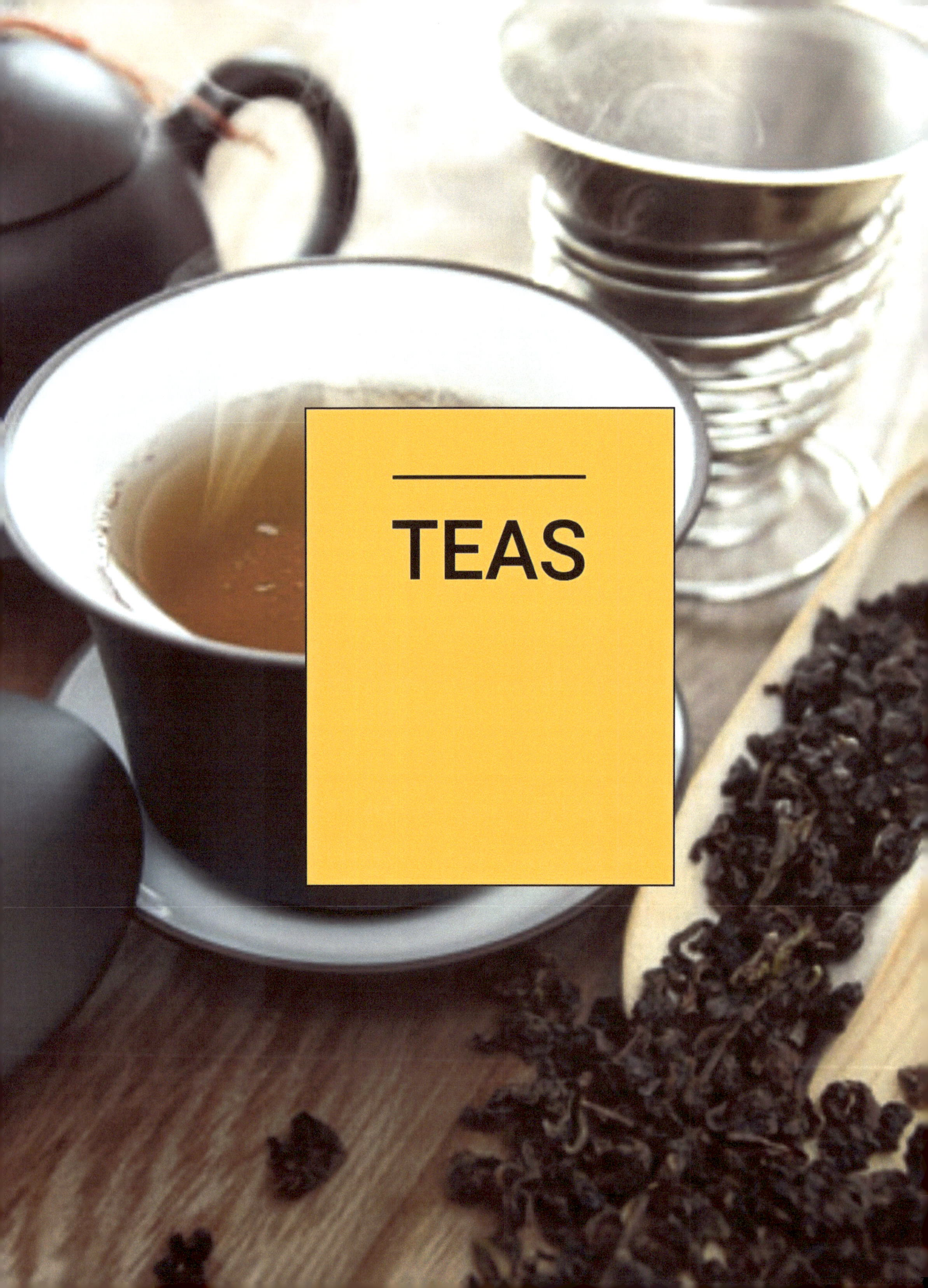
TEAS

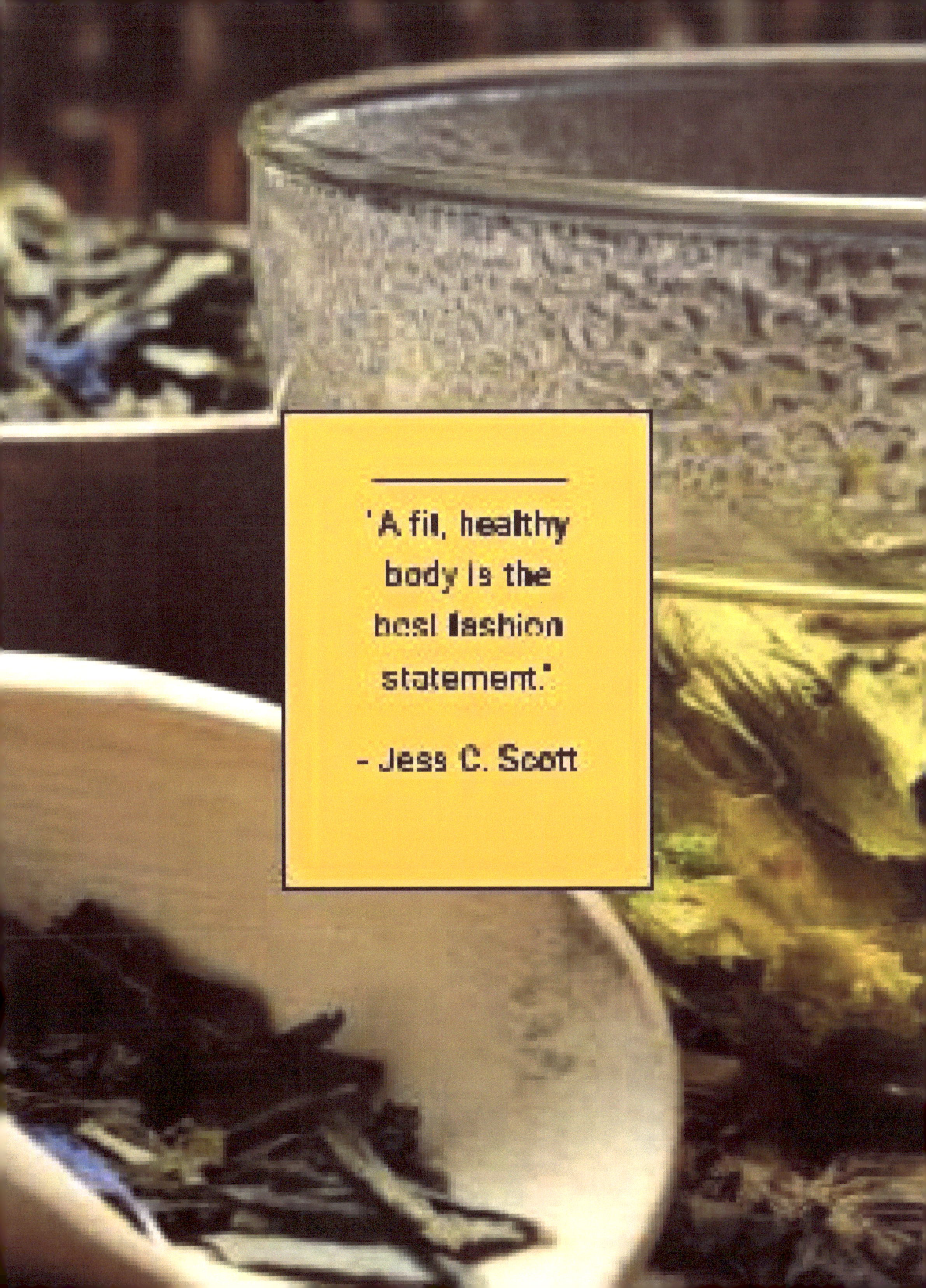
'A fit, healthy
body is the
best fashion
statement.'

- Jess C. Scott

TEAS FOR AILMENTS

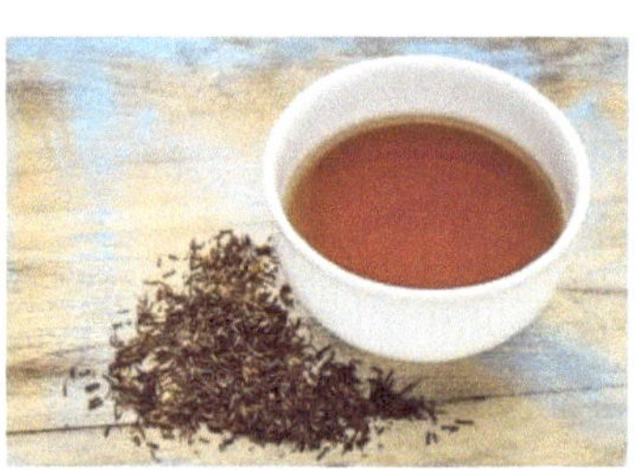

Rooibos Tea

- Naturally caffeine-free
- Soothes skin irritation
- Has cancer fighting properties

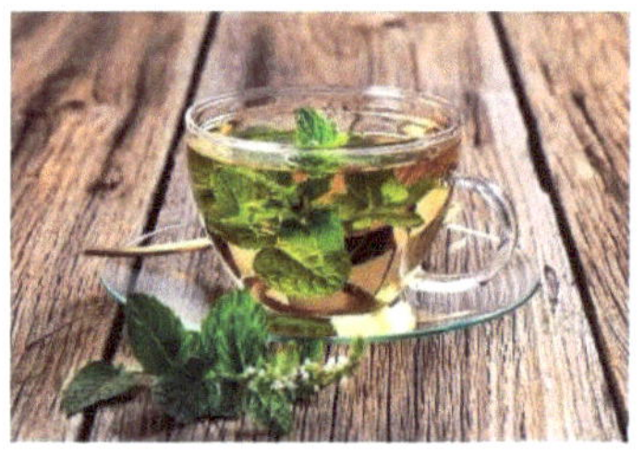

Peppermint Tea

- Decongestant
- Anti-inflammatory
- Suppresses the appetite

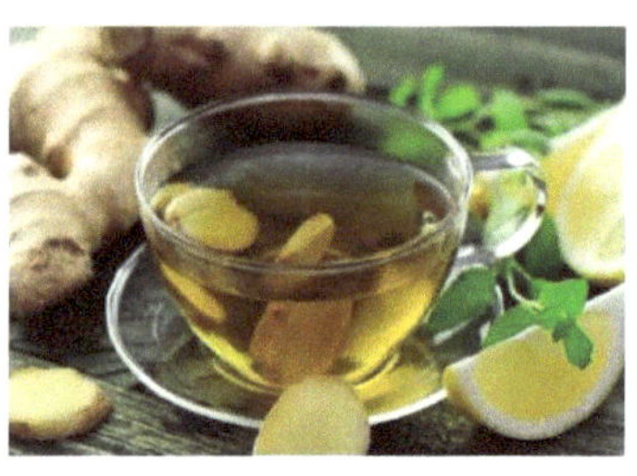

Dried Ginger Tea

- Has antihistamine properties
- Anti-inflammatory
- Eases motion sickness and nausea
- Flavor booster

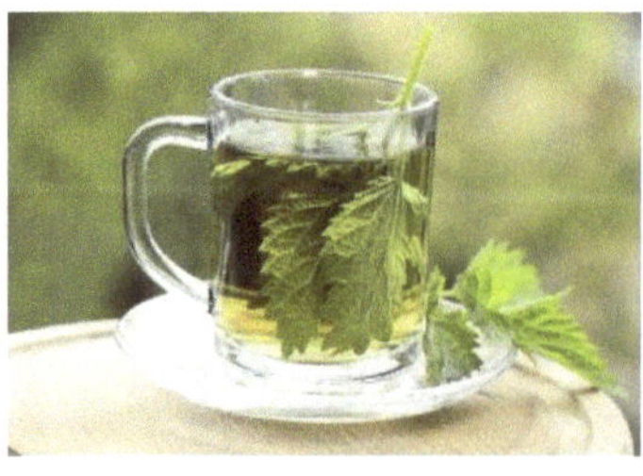

Stinging Nettle Tea

- Soothes seasonal allergies
- Energy booster
- Treats arthritis

TEAS FOR AILMENTS (CONT.)

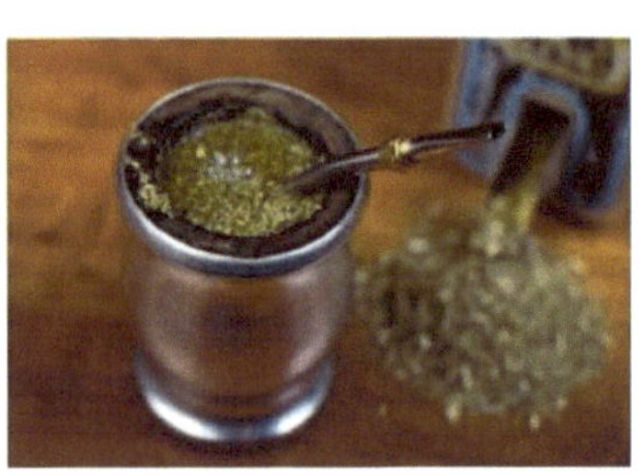

Yerba Mate Tea

- Opens up respiratory passages
- Reduces cholesterol and lowers blood pressure

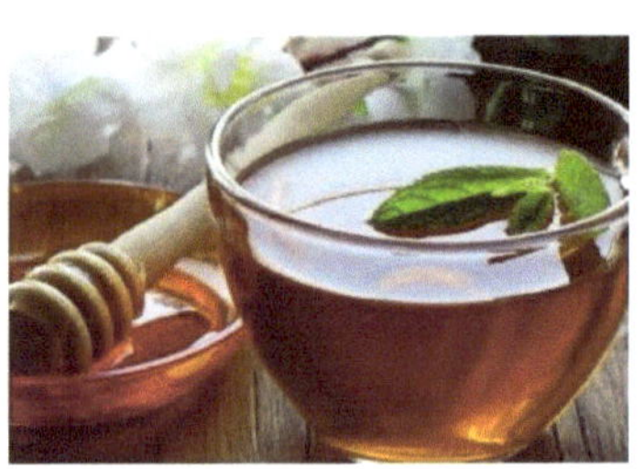

Lemon Balm Tea

- Has calming effects
- Helps with the common cold
- Helps with respiratory issues
- Regulates the digestive system
- Treats headaches and toothaches

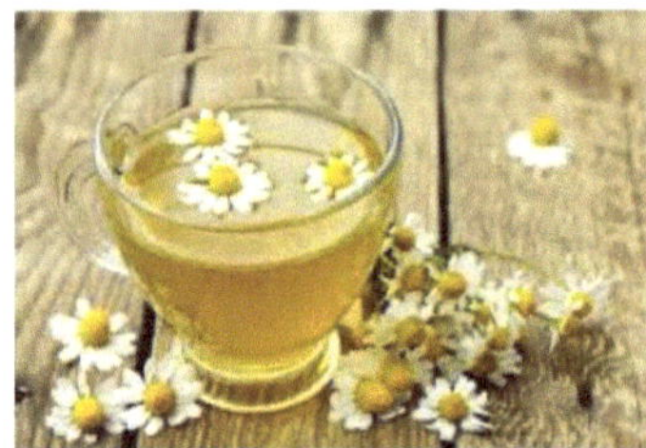

Chamomile Tea

- Antibacterial
- Treats stomach issues
- Promotes sleep

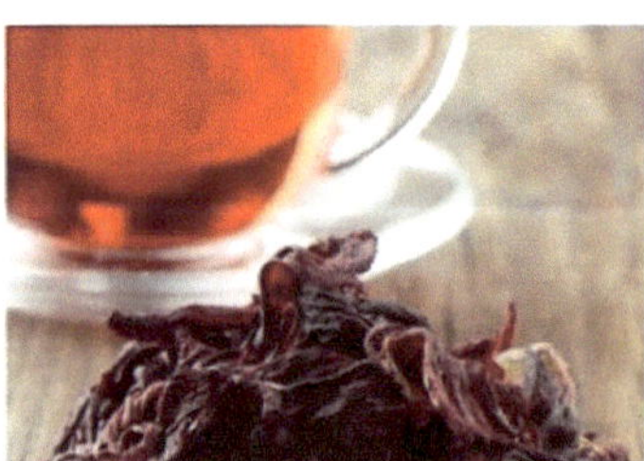

Hibiscus Tea

- Diuretic
- Lowers blood pressure
- Packed with vitamins

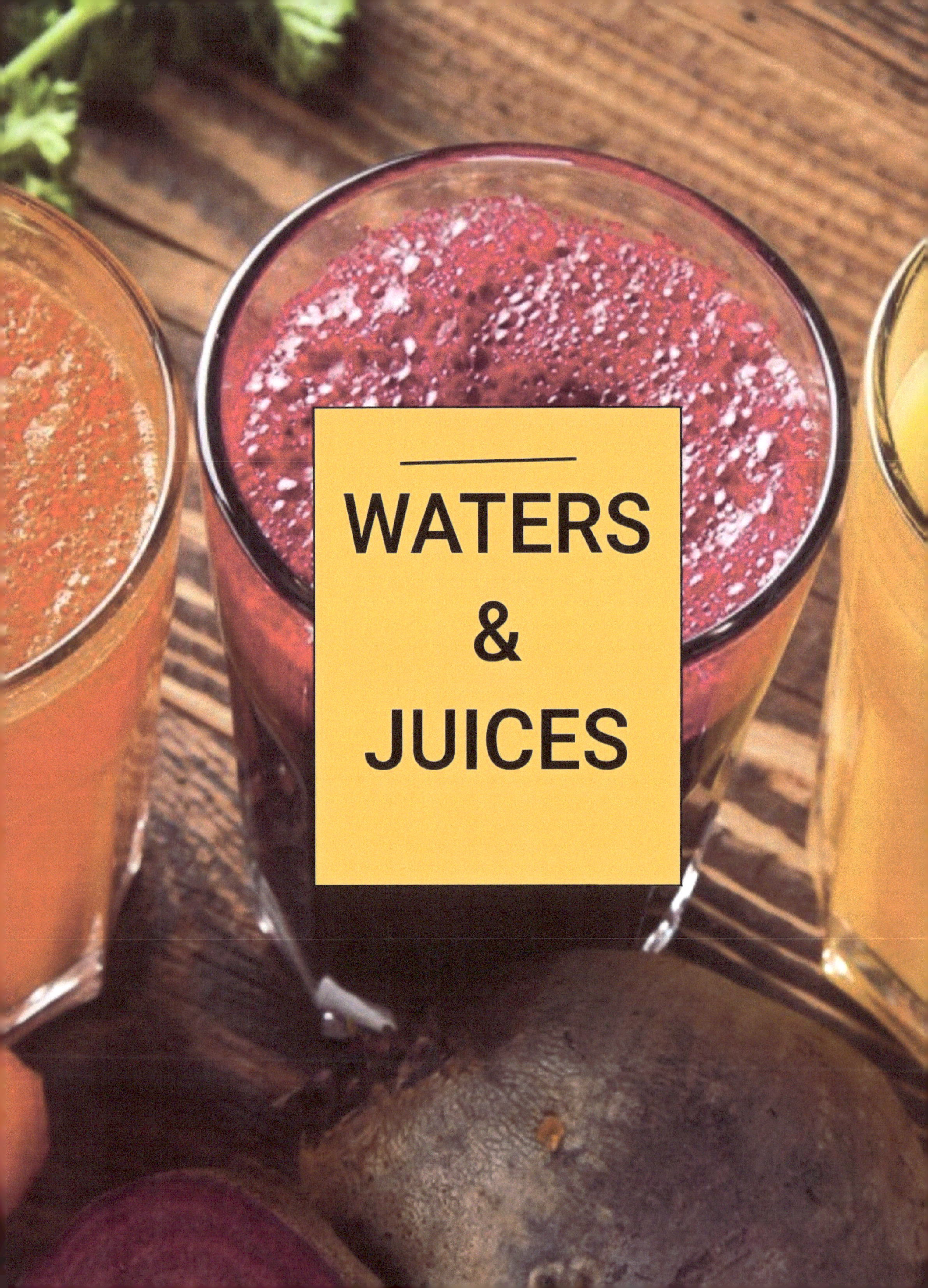

WATERS
&
JUICES

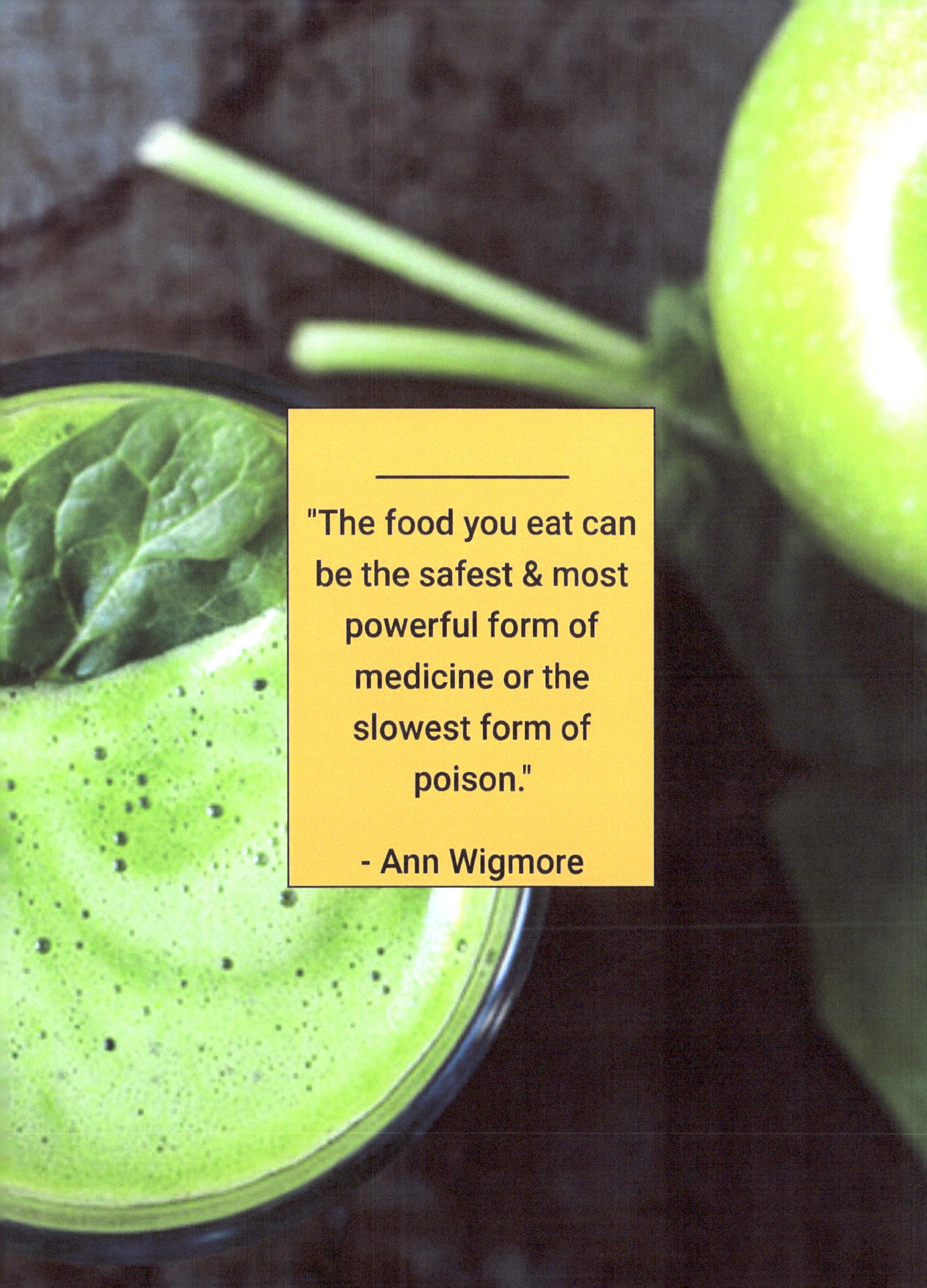
"The food you eat can be the safest & most powerful form of medicine or the slowest form of poison."

- Ann Wigmore

HELPFUL HINTS (CONT.)

Juices for ailments:

1. For a smoother consistency, water can always be added to each juice.
2. If needed, increase or decrease the amount of a certain fruit and/or vegetable.
3. Using organic fruits and vegetables ensures that your food holds significantly higher amounts of antioxidants. .

Water for weight-loss and detoxification:

1. Place all ingredients at the bottom of your pitcher, glass, or jar.
2. Cover your ingredients halfway with ice.
3. Top with water (preferably alkaline).
4. Place in the fridge for 1 - 2 hours before serving.
5. The container can be refilled at least 2 or 3 times with water before it loses its flavor.
6. Using organic fruits and vegetables ensures that your food holds significantly higher amounts of antioxidants.

If you, or someone you know, experiences discomfort
while detoxing, it is suggested to terminate the process.
There may be ingredients you need to add or leave out.
LISTEN TO YOUR BODY!

WATERS & JUICES (CONT.)

WATER	INGREDIENTS	USAGE
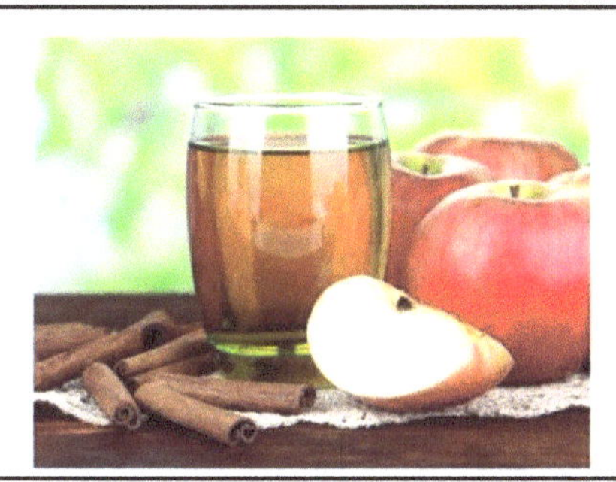	1 apple, 1 cinnamon stick	This combination boosts your metabolism, and helps fight against cancer, hypertension, diabetes, and heart disease. Additionally, ailments such as arthritis can bw soothed.
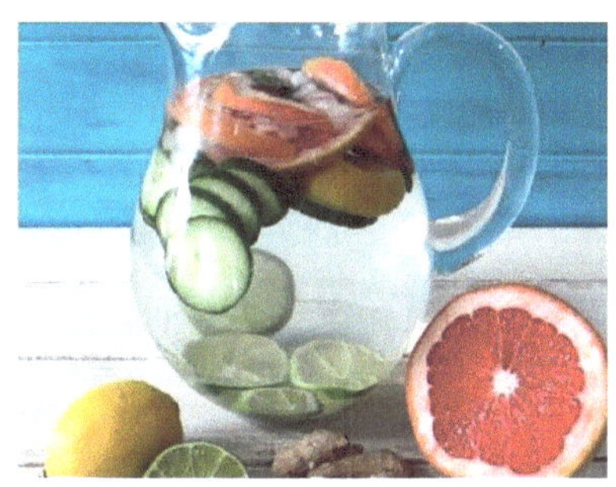	1/2 lemon (sliced), 1/2 lime (sliced), 1/2 grapefruit (sliced), 1 cup cucumber (cliced)	If you want to boost your metabolism and rid your body of toxins, drink at least a half a gallon for 3 - 5 days. Discard your pitcher of water after 24 hours.
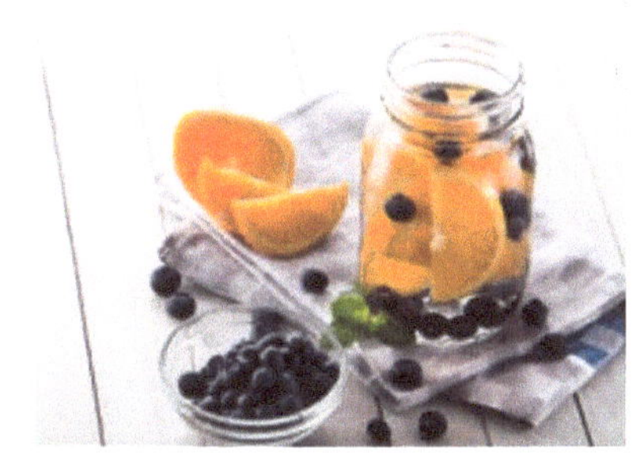	2 mandarin oranges, 1/2 cup of blueberries	To add more flavor to this mixture, squeeze the juice of an extra orange into the infused water. This combination aids in bone growth, and great for the immune system. Replenishes nutrients after menopause.
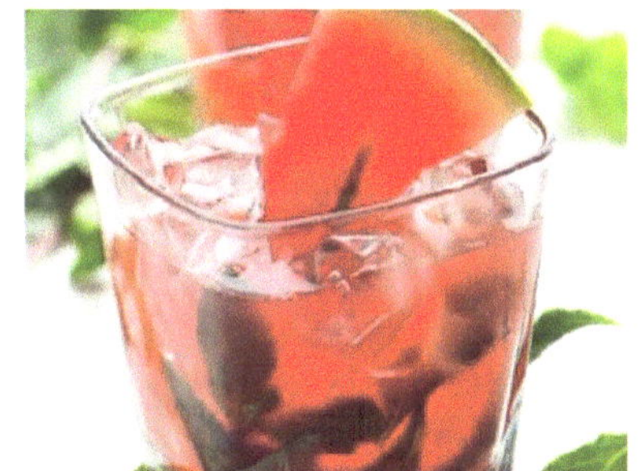	1/2 cup of strawberries, 4 cups of watermelon, 6 spring mint (crushed)	This combination helps boost metabolism, lower blood pressure, and soothes the muscles.
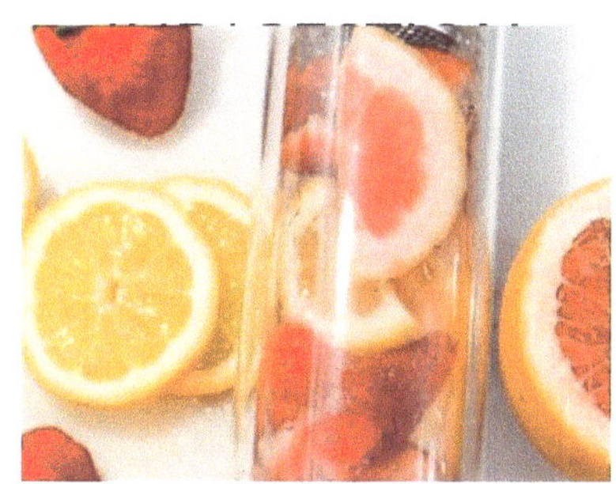	1 whole cucumber (thinly sliced), 2 cups fresh strawberries, 2 whole grapefruits (sliced), mint leaves (to taste)	This mixture helps burn belly fat and reduce the amount of starch found in the body. Additionally, this combination has anti-inflammatory properties.

WATERS & JUICES (CONT.)

WATER	INGREDIENTS	USAGE
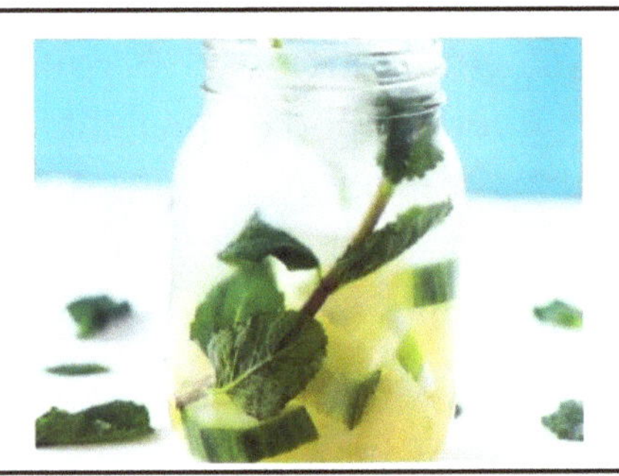	1 lemon (cut into wedges), 1/2 pineapple (cut into wedges), 2 limes (squeezed), few parsley leaves	This combination holds high doses of bromelain , which helps your metabolism break down proteins.
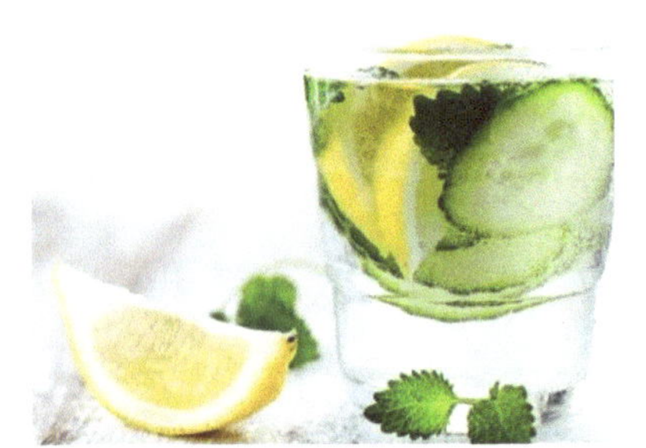	1 cucumber (sliced), 2 inches of ginger root (peeled), 2 lemons (cut into wedges), 10 fresh mint leaves	This mixture helps reduce the swelling of the stomach, helps burn fat, helps digestion, and aids in the prevention of gas and inflammation.
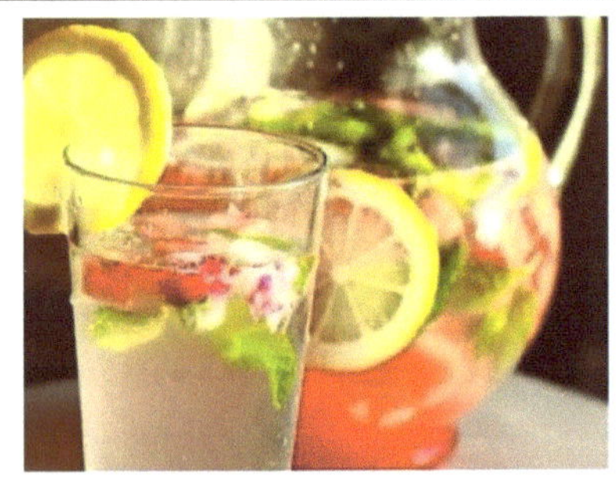	1 cup of watermelon (cut into cubes), 1 lemon, 1 orange, 1/2 cucumber	Squeeze half of the juice from the lemon and the orange into the water. Cut the remainder of the fruit into pieces, and add in the watermelon and cucumber slices. Great for the skin and weight management.
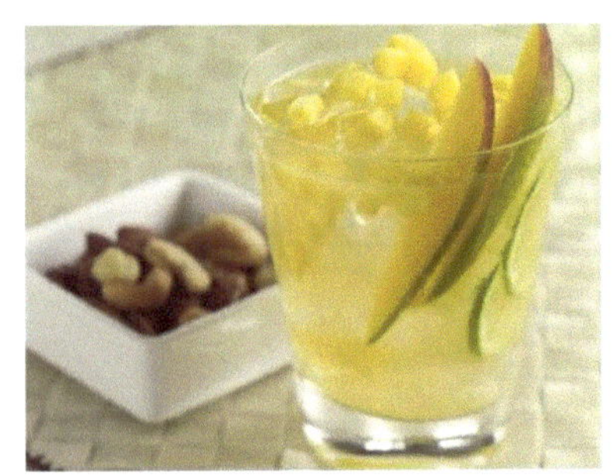	1 cup mango (cut into cubes), 1 inch ginger root (peeled and sliced)	This combination helps boost metabolism, eases migraines, menstrual cramps, heartburn, boosts memory, increases sex drive, and helps with digestion.
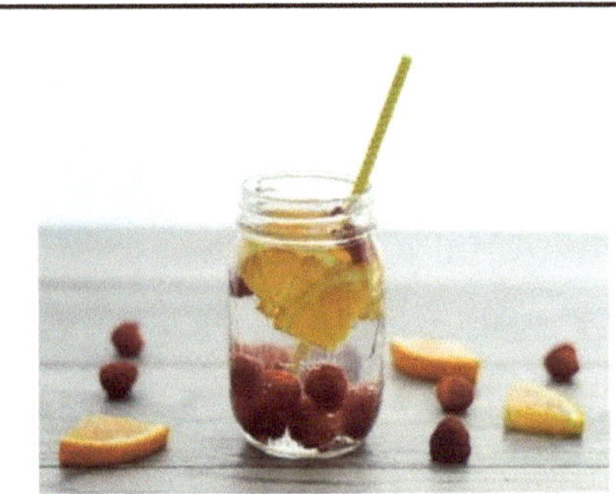	1 orange (thinly sliced), 1 cup of raspberries (lightly crushed)	This water is packed with Vitamin C, helps fight inflammation, and works against aging.

WATERS & JUICES (CONT.)

WATER	INGREDIENTS	USAGE
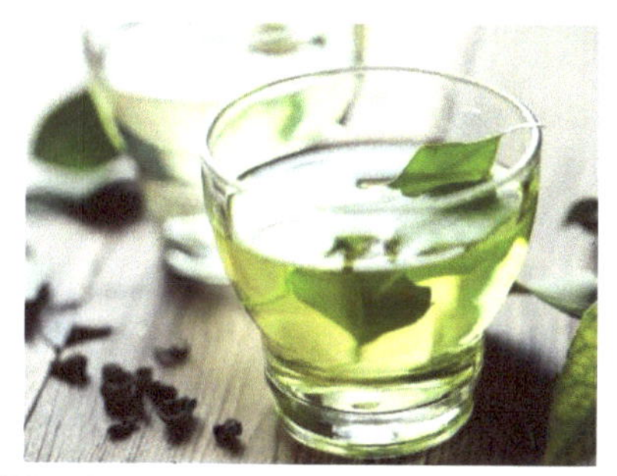	1 cucumber (peel ed and sliced)	This simple infusion is used to re-hydrate the skin and body, fight acne, and overall revitalize the body system.
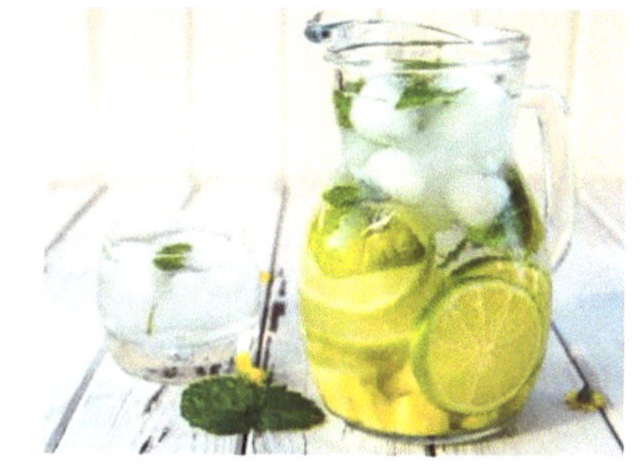	1 - 2 stalks of rosemary, 1 - 2 dried oregano leaves, 1/2 cucumber (thinly sliced), 1 cup kiwi (cut into cubes)	This combination will level up your detox experience. With a slight spicy kick, this detox is great for skin conditions, urinary tract issues, and helps aid in digestion.
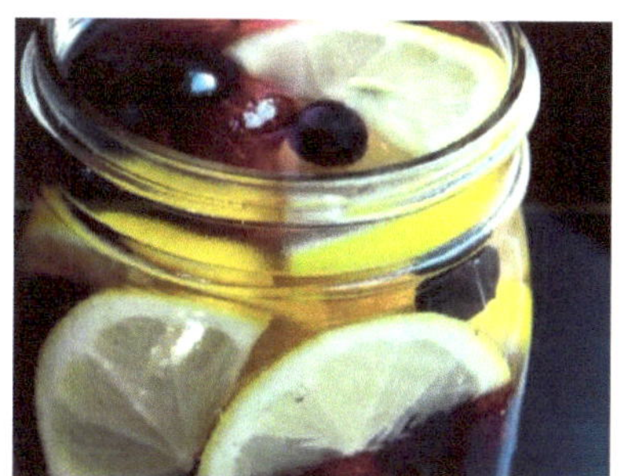	1 apple (thinly sliced), 2 oranges (cut into wedges), 2 pinches of rosemary, a dash of Himalayan salt	This herbal mixture will leave a sweet taste in your mouth while fighting against boosting energy, increasing metabolism, and eliminating toxins from the body.
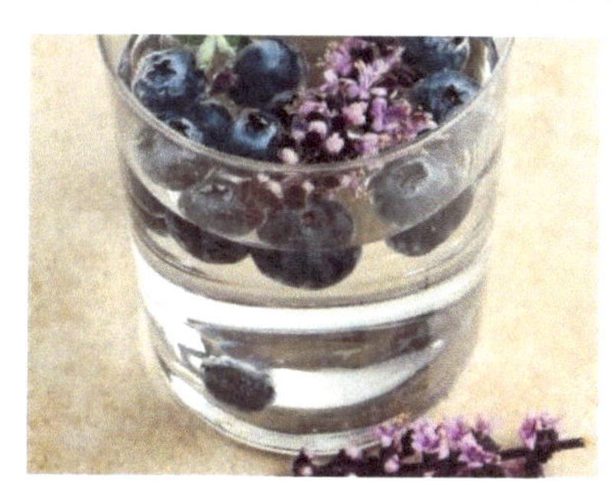	1 lemon (thinly sliced), 1/2 cup blueberries, 1/2 cup of raspberries	This infused water helps boost the immune system and promotes healthy skin.
	1 cup of blueberries, 1/4 cup of lavender leaves	This combination brings about calmness and relaxation. It also flushes out the system, calms an upset stomach, and boosts the immune system.

WATERS & JUICES (CONT.)

WATER	INGREDIENTS	USAGE
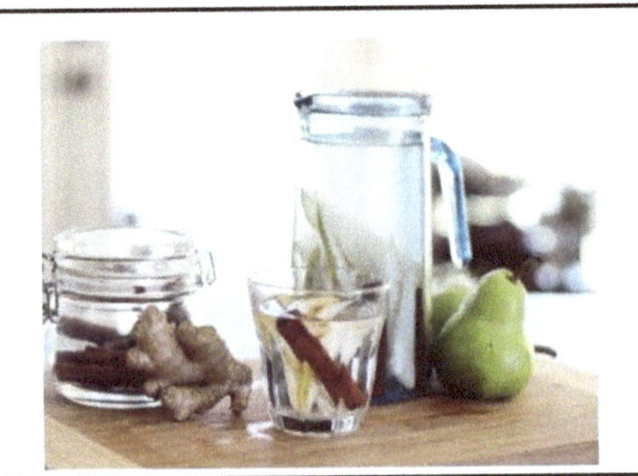	2 pears (cut into cubes), 2 lemons (cut into wedges), 1/2 orange (squeezed), handful of fresh basil leaves	This mixture if high in fiber, and will re-hydrate the body. Additionally, it is a great immune booster.
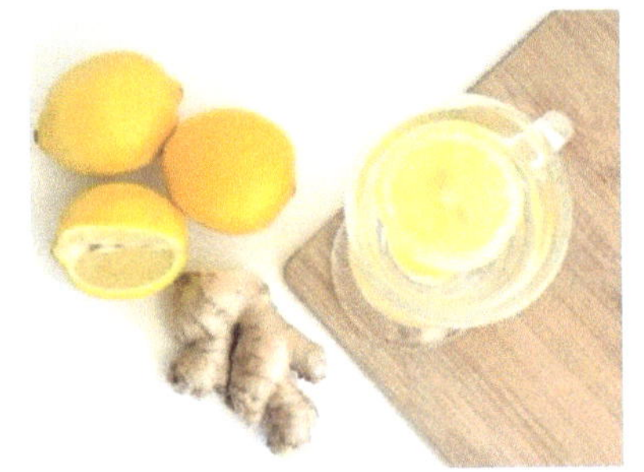	3 lemons, 1 inch ginger roots (peeled), 1 tablespoon of ground red chili powder	Squeeze two lemons into the infused water, and cut the third into wedges. This is a great immune booster and rich in antioxidants.
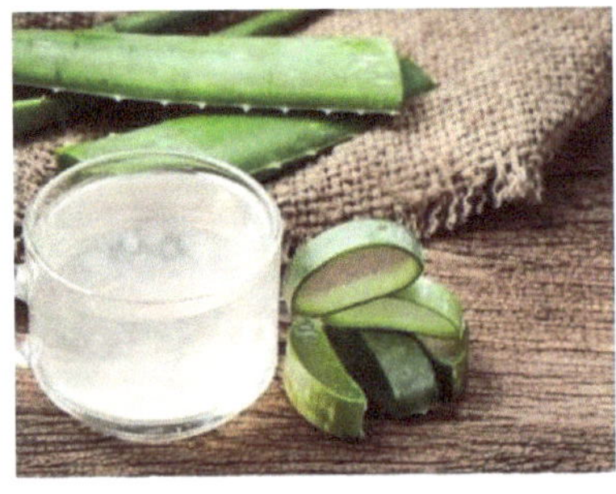	2 oranges (sliced), 1 lemon (squeezed), 1/4 inner leaf aloe vera gel, mint leaves to taste	This combination helps rid the body of toxins and manage body weight
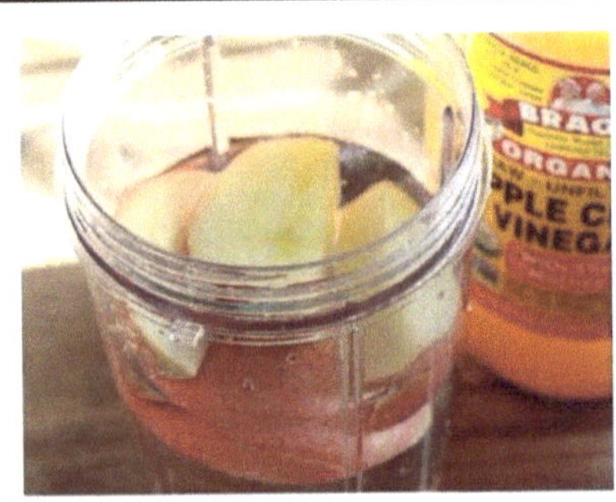	2 tablespoons of apple cider vinegar (ACV), 1 lime (sliced), 1 lemon (sliced), 5 - 6 mint leaves	This infused combination eliminates toxins and promotes healthy weight loss. Check with your physician if you are currently on blood thinners, diuretoics, and insulin.

HEALTH IS NOT ABOUT THE WEIGHT YOU LOSE, BUT ABOUT THE LIFE YOU GAIN!

DECIDE. COMMIT. SUCCEED.

- http://www.forkstofeet.com/2016/08/15-body-cleansing-fruits.html
- https://www.shape.com/blogs/weight-loss-coach/8-dos-donts-detoxing
- https://draxe.com/detox-bath-recipes/
- http://www.health.com/nutrition/planning-a-detox-or-juice-cleanse-5-dos-and-donts
- https://www.mindbodygreen.com/0-8404/top-10-reasons-to-detox-when-you-do-it-right.html
- http://helloglow.co/ginger-detox-bath/
- http://www.primallyinspired.com/friday-favorites-lavender-eucalyptus-bath-soak/
- https://www.laurengreutman.com/detox-bath-recipe/#_a5y_p=1768661
- https://www.thehappierhomemaker.com/homemade-milk-bath-recipe/
- http://mylifeandkids.com/simple-diy-almond-milk-bath/#_a5y_p=2543423

- https://tidymom.net/2013/lemon-rosemary-bath-salts-recipe/
- http://omnomally.com/2013/08/24/home-made--backpain-bath-salts/
- http://helloglow.co/the-health-benefits-of-tea-15-teas-for-any-ailment/
- http://www.theindianspot.com/effective-juice-cures-for-common-problems/
- http://www.behappyforlife.net/soak-feet-natural-bath-eliminate-toxins-body/
- http://7-min.com/slim-down-detox-water-with-cucumber-lemon-and-grapefruit/
- https://www.loseweightbyeating.com/apple-cinnamon-water-recipe/
- https://sunshinesouthern.wordpress.com/2013/04/27/green-tea-detox-bath/
- http://www.thepeachkitchen.com/2013/07/blueberry-%E2%99%A5-orange-water-infuse-your-water/

- http://www.valleymagazinepsu.com/weighing-in-6-delicious-detox-waters-to-cleanse-your-body-and-brighten-your-life/
- http://7-min.com/lemon-berry-infused-water/
- https://www.thedailymeal.com/healthy-eating/these-are-healthiest-fruits-infuse-your-water
- http://www.superskinnyme.com/ginger-lemon-detox-water-recipe.html
- https://www.livestrong.com/article/76566-apple-cider-vinegar-detox-diet/

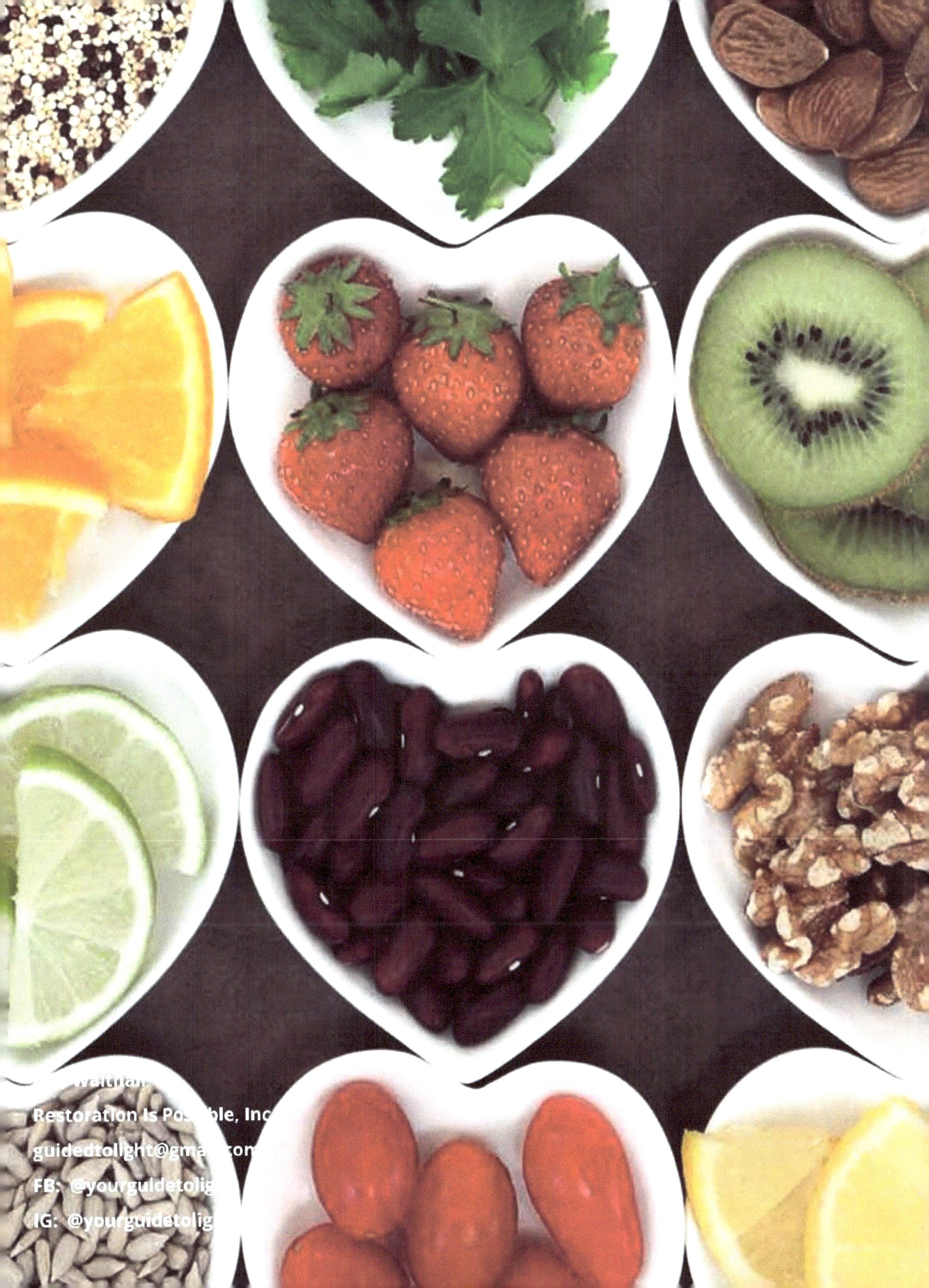
Waltham
Restoration Is Possible, Inc.
guidedtolight@gmail.com
FB: @yourguidetolight
IG: @yourguidetolight

www.ingramcontent.com/pod-product-compliance
Lightning Source LLC
Chambersburg PA
CBHW040150240726
48664CB00002B/646